Do Something!

Get Active!

By Tanisha Cook

ISBN 978-1-105-30844-4

FOREWORD

Some form of activity or recreation should be a part of every ones lives.

It makes you feel good and makes you look good all at the same time.

There is nothing like exercise, health and wellbeing. Your health outweighs everything else in your life. So why not increase your lifespan in a way that you will enjoy doing so.

Recreations are enjoyable, not torturing. Find an activity and do it with laughter and fun.

You may have pounds to loose or none at all, but the whole point is to enjoy your life while you still have air in your lungs.

The temple <u>you are in</u> belongs to the Father and no one else. Take care of it and enjoy and watch your body transform. As your body transforms, your mind will transform into a better you.

You will find a new person that wasn't there before or someone that you haven't met before, but have lost contact with along the way by not having time for him or her.

You are your best friend. You are who makes you laugh and cry. In a life of tribulations, who wants to seek more misery? You have one life and make it count.

If you have a family, recreations will help you get closer to them. It's not expensive to do most of the recreations listed; I guarantee it will be well within your budget.

And if it's well within your budget, you definitely have nothing to lose.

PREFACE

I know this book will touch you in the same way it touched me when I was writing it.

My research opened my eyes as well. There are other things to do in this life than just work.

Get some recreation and enjoy the fruits of your labor.

I thank the Father who has created all things and especially you.

New Jersey, 2011
Tanisha Cook, Author

Do Something!

Get Active

Table of Contents

Page

Introduction

This is a fast paced society. In this day and age, poverty has stricken many homes in America and around the world.

The need to indulge in an activity is far from many people's minds. They need to wake up and see that life is more than just hurts, but joy.

Recreation means to amuse or to stimulate yourself in a way that pleases you. Creation means to create something into existence. Recreate yourself while doing something with your body that will be beneficial to your <u>mind</u> and <u>spirit</u>.

A part of you that's willing to do something else is screaming out of many of us, but we don't hear the voice.

People are busy with their lives at the point where they have been doing the same thing over and over again for years and **without** happiness.

Happiness is something that you must acquire. You must want it. If you are too busy for it, then it will pass you by.

Recreating yourself through exercise or activity for a few extra hours a week is a sneeze if you feel that you will make it to the age of 100.

On that note, many seniors are into recreations to prolong their lives.

It never too late and you're never too old to take part in recreations, so do something.

Recreations I take Part of

I love to stay active and take part in different recreations. I do them by myself or with my family.

I take part in bicycling, Hiit Workouts and spinning classes, swimming volleyball, running, dance, playing with my children & pets and also roller skating. I love to go shopping and I find some fun out of doing housework.

All of my children have bicycles and we ride up and down our block when it's nice outside. I work up a sweat as do my children.

We stop and start again and within an hour I want to relax while my children ride for hours more.

I love to do High Intensity Interval training. I take part in this recreation at home in front of the television or at the gym. The gym supplies the spinning classes which are truly fun and rewarding at the end. The rest of my day after doing these recreations have me buzzing around like a bumble bee who is trying to find the right flower.

When it is hot I like to swim at the beach and when it's cold out, I like to swim indoors at the gym. The pool is kept warm and all you want to do is stay inside.

I play volleyball when I can. It's a favorite of mines. I believe I would have to buy a net and play in my backyard when the spring time comes back around.

I feel light when I run and sweat a lot. I run around the oval track near my residence. When you run ladies, make sure that you have a secure fitness bra. At one point I bought mines too big.

Dancing is a love of mines. I dance to worship & praise music. It's soothing and refreshing. As I dance, I know the Father is pleased with me.

Playing with my children and pets is a down time for me. I am reconnecting with my children as we interact, knowing that they will be children for a short time. I take that time out for them. My moments with them are full of laughter.

When I play with my dogs they pounce and my cats purr when I entertain them. They love my rub downs, especially my Boots, who is my huge 11 month old cat.

Roller-skating will never leave me. I prefer the normal roller skates, not the in line. Roller skating works the large muscle groups in my legs. The more you exercise them, the more calories you burn. It is true that you can be cellulite free.

What does the Holy Scriptures say?

The Holy Scriptures doesn't say much about exercise, besides exercising your mind to do the things of the Messiah.

But refuse profane and old wives fables, and exercise thyself

rather unto godliness.

For bodily exercise profiteth little: but godliness is profitable unto all things,

having promise of the life that now is, and of that which is to come.

This is a faithful saying and worthy of all acceptation.

1st Timothy 4:7-9

Pause...this doesn't mean not to exercise. This scripture means that exercising the body is less important than your spiritual walk. If you live holy it will be profitable to you.

But seek ye first the kingdom of God, and his righteousness;

and all these things shall be added unto you.

Matthew 6:33

If you seek to do some form of recreation, it would be best if you have Jesus on your side. When you have HIM, you have everything.

We know that Jesus and the disciples walked many miles. We also know that keeping God's temple healthy is important.

What? Know ye not that your body is the temple of the Holy Ghost which is in you, which ye have of God, and ye are not your own?

For ye are bought with a price: therefore glorify God in your body, and in your spirit, which are God's.

1st Corinthians 6:19-20

Don't you want to keep your body fit, so you won't have to feel your age?

Or do you want to be like this King;

...Eglon King of Moab: and Eglon was a very fat man.

Judges 3:17

There's more to this story about him being fat, but if you read on, you will see that if he wasn't fat he might have lived.

When you are fat or obese there could be many different reasons why, but the main reason is taking far too many calories that you weren't able to burn off throughout the day.

I eat a lot of the good things and take in less calories and I burn them all throughout the day. So my weight is roughly the same when I get on the scale weekly or monthly.

I have pleasure in doing my recreations. When I feel pain I stop. Make sure your recreation is pleasurable so you can enjoy becoming fit and trim.

There are many ways to get your action on, your limbs moving, your blood rushing and your heart pumping.

It takes 3 weeks to develop a habit, but for some... it takes much less.

1

<u>WEIGHT TRAINING</u>

What I love about weight training is the results right afterwards. My metabolism is up and my body is sore and I love it.

Most recreations give the same results, but the soreness of working those various muscles stands out from the rest.

I don't like the pain, but I do like the results after the soreness goes away.

To lift weights it is best to work with a personal trainer at first or you can get injured. No one wants a muscle tear. If not taken care of properly it can last for years...I know.

The specifics of weight training are found on various websites, books and also at your local gym, where there are weight training professionals.

2

<u>AEROBICS</u>

Aerobic exercise, who can forget the Jane Fonda age and how aerobic exercise has gone mad in a good way?

The list of channels and DVD's devoted to exercising your heart and burning calories is endless.

When doing aerobics there is soreness, but not as much for those who are used to it. You've just ripped your muscle fibers, as in weight training, and they need time to heal, so take some time off.

Aerobic exercisers use weights, balls, steppers etc. There is a wide range.

There is dance aerobics which I love and doing aerobics in the water is beneficial to seniors who are regaining their strength.

Aerobic exercisers range from beginners, intermediate and advancers and it will be wise to go slow. Many beginners seem to injury their knees most often. I did myself when I first started.

There is no need to jump around, just to keep it moving.

3

<u>RUNNING/JOGGING</u>

Running and Jogging are similar. Jogging is a slower pace and running can be fast and slow; depending on the person.

This easy recreation is very low cost and you may have to change sneakers every 6 months or buy a new music CD, but that's all for the benefits you get by doing this addictive recreation as many runners say.

Indoor running tracks are at various YMCA's and some gyms. Outdoor running is what more people prefer.

Marathons are held all over the world and runners travel and see all the beautiful countries on this green earth. They make their living running in marathons.

Running is rewarding. Your body and your mind will love it. If this is a recreation that you choose, you'll see that there's nothing like the breeze softly caressing your face.

4

GETTING PHYSICAL WITH YOUR SPOUSE

Use Parental Discretion before reading

This is a very important recreation with your spouse. The more the happier for the both of you, if you don't have any problems.

You will not only shrink your fat cells, but you will shrink more fat cells while sleeping. Be careful on snacking after this activity.

The muscles that you work depend on the position of this activity.

More positions mean different muscles worked, which also means the more fit you'll be. Have you ever played Twister?

When the heightened point comes during this activity, you will not only be burning with passion, but also burning calories.

5

<u>HOUSEWORK</u>

Not a daunting task if you want to have a sanitized home.

I enjoy house work by doing a number of things, like buying my favorite cleaning supplies and fragrances and then kicking everyone out the house (husband included), and putting on my favorite music.

I usually start with the living room and work my way up to the bathroom. My children can take care of their own rooms, but there are times when I do a spring cleaning to get the old clothes, papers and toys out the way.

Every season starts a new clean up. It's also a time for <u>goodwill</u> giveaways and I don't mean to the store. There are needy folks that will benefit from your housework, so in turn, you are helping yourself and helping others.

6
<u>FLOOR EXERCISES</u>

The effortless way to tone up while watching your favorite program is by sitting on your exercise mat or towel and doing stretches and then exercising your body parts.

Sit-ups, pushups, leg lefts and even a stepper can push you easily into a 30 to 2 hour workout depending on the program you are watching.

You can use dumbbells and resistance bands to tone your muscles. If there are commercials you can walk up and down the stairs for 2 minutes.

Exercise equipment and floor exercises go hand and hand. If you have watched infomercials before, you know what I mean.

Many people have the same fitness equipment stuffed in their closet collecting dust and making a special habitat for small leggy creatures. Some people who bought exercise equipment had lost the thrill of using it.

If you don't have equipment go to www.marshaghughes.com – Your body is your Gym.

7

HANG GLIDING

A recreation that I wouldn't mind trying in the future, but I know it would be a dare for most.

Being afraid of heights is a fear that doesn't have me locked down.

The first principle of hang gliding is to learn how to fly to see if this is for you. If you like it, you will have to purchase a hang glider. A good one is priced at $4,000.

It takes up to 6 months to learn how to do this recreation and there is no license required. But your instructor must be certified by the United States Hang Gliding Association.

To take part of this sport you must have strength, because you have to have balance and endurance.

8

<u>TENNIS</u>

The ball and the large racket are your instruments to help you win against your opponent that's on the other side of the long net that stretches from one end to the court to the other.

Your feet will take you through the competition souring in the air and back and forth on the court's pavement trying to hit the ball within the allowed court lines. You will definitely get an all body workout. Have you seen the famous tennis sisters?

This sport supposedly originated in England in the 19th century, but others say France in the 12th century. Either way you look at it, you know it's here to stay.

9

HIIT WORKOUT (High Intensity Interval Training)

The Hiit workout is an exercise that can last up to 20-30 minutes. For beginners there is a split of doing,

30 seconds of Hiit followed by 90 seconds of Rest – 6 to 8 sets

Interval training is intense physical training that includes bursts of High Pulsing workouts with periods of resting. Many cardio workouts are included, like running and jumping robe. It's about starting and stopping when you have exhausted your energy stores and then starting back up in 30 to 60 seconds.

The Hiit workout was popularized in the 1990's by Arthur Jones the founder of Nautilus.

Most people who are trying to lose weight have a great advantage when using Hiit, because their rate of getting fit is increased in a short amount of time.

10

<u>CAMPING</u>

Camping in the outdoors to be close to nature, is as close that you can get to the wild lives of large and small creatures. Make sure the camping site that you go to has less of the large animals roaming around.

For camping you will need a tent for shelter. You can bring dehydrated or canned foods or you can simply go hunting for it. If you do this you will need a fishing pool or a shotgun. Moving on...

To get your tent up you will need rope, stakes, a hammer and a broom for dusting. Most people that camp have a sleeping bag or use a twin size air mattress with a manual pump.

Don't forget the necessities of paper products. For less garbage you can purchase a camping dishware set for under 20 dollars.

For cleaning, soap and water is a much needed necessity. If you run out you can always go to the nearby creek or a general store that could be miles away. Don't forget to bring a change of clothes and personal hygiene products.

For a list of camping sites near you, go to www.reserveamerica.com

11

SPINNING

If you've ever rode a bike or never have, the only way you'll fall off this exercise bike is from depleting your energy stores and becoming totally exhausted.

My first class lasted fifty-five minutes long and I sweated like I never sweat before. The lights were out and colorful lights whipped around the room to the music.

The instructor in the front of the class encouraged everyone to stay focused and to lower their resistance on the bike to keep up with the class.

Spinning is a vigorous workout that burns many calories and keeps you in shape. You have to push yourself.

There is a DVD on spinning so you can do this recreation in your home, without going to the gym. Google it

12

JUMP ROPE

As a little girl I always enjoyed jumping rope. Double Dutch was my community's favorite in the late 70's.

If you could jump fast you were good and everyone wanted you. But if you couldn't turn those ropes, the girls didn't use you. I was bad at turning. I remember being scooted to play with the inexperienced girls, who normally had a terrible rope. It was something made out of hard wire.

The speed of jumping is not important, but how you handle the ropes come from wrist action. You grasp the handles and pull it towards your chest and begin with a good speed. Jump ropes can cost anywhere from 20 dollars.

A great jump rope workout is 15 minutes long, resting between 30 to 60 seconds and then doing 3 minutes of continuous jumping.

13
SHOPPING

This great recreation and workout can be done whether you have money or not. I know having money helps, but working a mall that's blocks long can burn calories plus you can compare prices for savings.

The wrong side of shopping is doing it while eating the wrong things from the mall restaurants and food stands.

Your shopping experience could last between 1 to 3 hours while you walk off unwanted pounds. You can burn up to 600 calories an hour depending on your current weight.

A pedometer can help you keep track of your steps. They are very cheap and under 5 dollars.

14
BASKETBALL

If you have a good basketball net and loose clothing, then you have everything you need to start this high intensity recreation.

I've never seen any overweight players on the High School, College or Professional basketball teams.

This sport consists of jumping, running and dribbling the ball. All of your muscle groups are at play as you score by playing a single game or with other players.

Some aerobic exercises implement the jump shot throw and the shuffle technique.

Playing basketball is fun and you will get a drizzle of sweat in no time.

15
BASEBALL - Exercises

Running, catching and swinging the bat is all a part of baseball sport's athletics. Instead of describing how to play this recreation, I'm going to outline the exercises that baseball players use to strengthen their athletic abilities.

*Speed training increases speed and endurance
*Hammer curls strengthen the arms
*Swiss ball exercises strengthens the lower and upper body
   (Other names – sports ball, exercise ball, Pilates
   ball, fitness ball and   stability ball)
*Side Planks help the abdominals and the back
   (To do planks, you position your body to do a
   pushup. Instead of your hands on the floor your
   forearms will rest on the floor. You hold the

position and contract your abs and hold for 30 seconds and then repeat, doing 3-5 reps)

Baseball players don't need to build muscle mass, but strength. They must give the muscle group that they have worked on 1 to 2 days to recover.

Strengthening your body as they do will help you hit a home run every time.

16

<u>FOOTBALL - Exercises</u>

Football is played in different ways in different countries and more than just a 2 person game. In this chapter I'll talk about the football exercises so you can gain muscle strength.

Football exercises are the bench press, bicep curls, abdominal workouts and neck exercise using neck resistance. (You do this exercise by sitting in a chair. You wrap a small towel around the back of your head. You hold the ends and move your head in an up and down motion)

*The Bench Press helps your chest muscles get stronger
*Doing Bicep curls helps your arms gain strength
*Abdominal workouts help the core of your whole body in balance
*Pull ups helps you gain upper body strength. (You grab an overhead bar   with both of your hands and lift your body towards it)

The game of football includes a lot of running, catching and tackling. Something many of us do every day. Think about it.

17
<u>TRACK</u>

Running track on the oval rubber pavement, road running, cross country and racing are some of the athletics done on the track.

Athletes sprint, run hurdles, participate in middle and long distance running, the long jump, throws, relays and the Pole vault.

Most schools take part in track sports. A student can win a scholarship for college and a person can make a career taking part of different sports on the track.

As a former resident of Bronx New York, I used to run on the track across the street from Yankee stadium, since then the track now harbors the new Yankee stadium.

I wonder where the city is going to put another.

18

<u>VOLLEYBALL</u>

This is one of my recreations. The competition of 2 people running and hitting the ball and using hand techniques is fun inside the park and on the beach.

The net used in volleyball is usually 32x3 feet long. The ball is light weight and comes in a variety of colors.

A team has 6 players with 3 on each side. The positions of these players are right back, right front, middle front, left front, left back and middle back.

The way you move your feet in playing this recreation is a very important aspect of the game. Before you jump, your arms are the leader. It propels you to jump high to hit the ball. Another key component is to always know where the ball is on the opposite side.

19

<u>SOCCER</u>

If you have a head you can play this game, a little humor.

This is a recreation that can cause headaches, which I'm not a fan of getting; but on the good side it is fun and it can turn you into a professional.

The basics of playing soccer are passing and throwing the ball, retrieving it from another player, dribbling and shooting it by using your head and tackling your opponent as a defense.

More than one person needs to play. A team of players are 11. It is known that to play soccer it will take you a bit of time to learn it. You must learn how to kick properly. Learning the different techniques can get confusing, but there are approaches that a coach can do to speed up your process.

For more on soccer organizations, go to www.ussoccer.com

20 ROLLERSKATING   21 ICE SKATING

22 SKATE BOARDING

I started roller skating and ice skating as a teenager and it's only something I do sparingly. Mama needs a new pair of skating shoes.

Skate boarding is my eldest son's recreation of choice.

- For those interested in Roller Skating, you should buy a high quality brand, because used can get you bruised.
- All forms of skating works the leg muscles and abdominals
- Most skating rinks are oval shaped and patrons roll to different kinds of the music
- Roller skating can be a form of transportation
- On roller skates you can jump, spin and do numerous acrobats

- The first roller skates had one wheel placed in the front and one wheel placed in the back of the shoe.

For those interested in Ice Skating

- Ice skating is more like roller skating except for the bottom of the shoe contains a metal blade that cuts along an icy pavement.
- Figure skating and other competitive sports are popular for using these shoes; Hockey, Tour skating, Brandy, Ringette and Short track.

For those interested in Skateboarding

- This flat oval shaped board with wheels underneath helps children and adults do tricks and help them travel.
- A long board is a longer skateboard that measures 84 to 150 centimeters long.
- Many professional skateboarders skate on ramps, concrete hills, participate in skating boarding competitions, where prizes and money are won.
- China has the largest skateboard park in the world.

23

<u>BICYCLING</u>

Bicycling or Cycling or just riding a bike is a recreation for all ages. Bicycles come in 1 wheel (unicycle), three (tricycle) or four wheels (quadricycles). Henry ford made the first quadricycle. How modern are they today?

Bikes can cost as low as fifty dollars and as high as two thousand. The better the quality, the more you are going to pay, but the cost doesn't outweigh the benefits.

For use as a recreation or travel, you will tone up your legs, abdominals and arms.

It has been known that your life span can increase by 15 to 20 years bicycling often.

Many people who own bikes boost their metabolism bicycling for an hour a day. You may want to start by riding on your days off and then riding to and from work in order to cut transportation cost.

Having a bike is low maintenance and your health can also be low maintenance if you take up a recreation like this one.

24

<u>KITE FLYING</u>

When someone tells you to go fly a kite, just say ok.

This soothing activity is definitely a day off recreation. There are different kites that you may want to purchase.

- Diamond for low/medium winds
- Delta for low/medium winds
- Dragon for low/medium winds
- Box and the Parafoil is for stronger winds

It depends on nature to do this recreation. Lightening and rain are the worst conditions to exercise your kite flying talents. Become a smart kite flyer.

There may be times when you need help propping your kite. When it's up in the air, stand with your back against the wind.

There is indoor Kite Flying and it can also be just as fun. You don't have to worry about the elements.

25

<u>DANCE</u>

Dancing is movement of the flow of the body. Dancing lifts your spirit and connects to your every being. Just about everyone on the planet Earth loves to dance in some fashion.

Mentioning the different dances will make this subject hundreds of pages long, so I'll keep it simple.

Dancing allows what you feel to come through quick or slow body movements. The use of your head, arms, waist, legs and feet are in play and grooving to the rhythms.

Some people dance by themselves, others in groups, some for competition and some to wind down after work, which is usually on a weekend.

The benefits of dancing are priceless. Whether there is music or not, you know what you feel in your heart.

26

PAINTING

One gift that's a treasure to have and that is the art of painting. An amateur or starving artist can make an impact using their artistic ability.

To get started you will need a canvas full of paper and paints and some know how in order to get a decent image.

There are many ways to paint, some people finger paint, spray paint and some use acrylic paints for a more tamed look.

There are many classes given in community colleges and centers and amateurs are always welcome.

The most painting I've done was finger painting as a young child. But it will be fun to do some serious painting one day.

27

<u>ROCK CLIMBING</u>

Rock climbing is a recreation that you probably couldn't get most to do.

It does require a lot of upper body strength. Whether indoors or outdoors rock climbing builds strong muscle and the gain of rock climbing techniques can lead you to climbing large mountains, if you want to go there.

Many amusement parks have them, so you can climb your way to the top of their rock climbing panels for minimal cost. There are also rock gyms.

A must for rock climbing is to be equipped with a harness and a carabine for attaching it to the rope you are using.

Other equipment needed – helmet, hand chalk, climbing shoes, quick draws and a belay device to create friction, it's like a brake so if the climber falls it will keep you from falling.

28

<u>GOLF</u>

This is not a boring recreation as some non-enthusiast say. This recreation requires a lot of thinking.

You need golf clubs, golf balls and a golfing location to do your swing thing.

The typical golf bag has 12 different clubs, the more clubs/tools you have the better you'll be able to play the game.

The gold clubs needed are 7 irons, 1 hybrid, 3 woods and a putter.

Woods hit long shots, hybrids is a combination of iron and wood. The irons are used for when you're less than 200 yards from the green.

Wedges are specialty irons and the putter gets the ball in the hole. A moment where we see golfers celebrate their win.

29

<u>HIKING</u>

You can hike alone or with your family. Hiking is pure exercise, fresh air with nature all around.

There are many places to hike in America. Trails could be woody landscapes, rocky mountains and difficult terrains.

You would want your hiking experience to last and it can with pictures, so bring your cameras.

For your hiking needs you will need a back pack full of the necessities.

- Canteen for your water or thirst quenching drink
- Sunscreen to protect you from harmful sun rays
- Binoculars
- A compass to know which direction you're traveling
- Your identification and your cell phone

Hiking for 2 to 4 hours is great outdoor recreation. If you develop pain, stop and engulf in the scenery of the open air.

For trails in your area, go to www.trails.com

30

SCUBA DIVING

It's nothing like being among the fishes. For those who like going in the ocean, this recreation can lead to an underwater experience, literally.

The best way to take part in scuba diving is in safe waters, especially for beginners. Their first experience shouldn't be a frightening one.

Professionals usually have a shark suit on which helps to prevent serious damage to the body. A pole spear is also used under water for hunting fish. Some scuba divers use it as a just in case weapon.

To begin your scuba diving, you must wear a wet suit, diving mask, boots, fins, goggles and an underwater camera for picture taking.

The oxygen tank which helps you breath underwater is 21% oxygen and full of compressed air.

Scuba diving is a must try for me. I'm hoping to go on vacation to take part in this recreation.

31

<u>SURFING</u>

Surfing isn't just for the Californians, but for us on the east coast too. Getting a surf board and learning balance will get you soaring among the waves.

Surfboards float on water and you can lay on it while you learn how to balance it in your pool or at the shallow end of the beach. If you put too much weight in the back of the board, you will twist overboard.

Paddling the board with one hand will help you gain consistent speed in order to catch a wave.

Standing on the board takes practice, but we know practice makes you a perfectionist at whatever you do.

Surfboards cost is usually $180 and up, which is affordable.

Buying a surfboard will be worth your while for fun in the sun and the waves.

32

<u>GARDENING</u>

Planting a large or small garden takes patience. The rewards are fresh and organic veggies & fruits if you don't use pesticides.

Gardening is easier when you buy the plants at a home improvement store. Planting seeds and waiting to see the tiny plant grow takes a toll on your patience, but you can say you've grown your crop from scratch, so to speak.

I garden almost every year in New Jersey, from vegetables to apple & peach trees in my backyard.

Indoor green houses come in all sizes and can fit inside a typical apartment.

33

<u>SWIMMING</u>

A recreation I love to do, with the help of a nose clip for my nose and goggles for my eyes to see underwater. I just haven't trained my eyes yet.

I've never been fond of bathing hats. I wear my hair natural, so if it's going to get wet, so be it.

Swimming exercise benefits are full of resistance against the water which you can take part in all year round.

Swimming activities are in many schools and someone can make a living from their athletic ability.

Here are different stroke techniques:

- The Freestyle
- Backstroke
- Breaststroke
- Butterfly

Learn more at www.usa.swimming.org.

34

<u>HORSEBACK RIDING</u>

I remember going to a Dude Ranch as a teenager and riding on a horse. I was a little scared, because of the bumpy terrain and the horse I was riding on kept turning his head to look at me and he had a continuing case of flatulence.

There was no one holding my horse. The professionals were leading the trail. It was one horse after another with my classmates riding horses as well.

I can tell you that I would like to do it again, but this time I need training. There are places in every state where you can learn how to horseback ride.

The attractiveness of this recreation is that if you are an experienced rider, you can train as an athlete and have a career.

Riding horses develops your coordination skills and helps you balance. Many muscles are being used including your legs, abdominals, shoulders and back. The faster you ride the more calories you burn. Riding is therapeutic and also helps with digestion.

35

<u>VIDEO GAMES</u>

Playing video games is a recreation that many children and adults love to enjoy. For myself, I prefer the thinking video games and the ones that get me up out of my seat and moving.

The Play stations, X-box's and Wiis are expensive, but the prices are lowering.

Video games have been around a long time. I clearly remember Atari with Pac man eating his power pellets. I thought it was annoying, but as we know the game is a true classic.

Video game recreation can last as long as you are interested in watching the screen and moving your limbs.

The bestselling video games are violent, because we live in a violent world. The worst ones just get tossed after a few seasons.

The biblical video games sales are slow, but they are about to establish major ground and the video games that get you moving are on the rise.

Dance, aerobics and bowling video games are helping people to lose weight, which most Americans need to do.

Moving your body while playing to win, is satisfaction to your physical and your mental state.

36

<u>HANDBALL</u>

When I was younger and living in the projects of the Bronx, we had a handball court in the community. It was always crowded. Competitors won money and losers continued to compete until they got it right or won their money back.

I played one time and my hand hurt, because my hand wasn't properly protected. You will need handball gloves that will help the force of the ball leave little impact in your palm.

Handball can be played by 2 or more people. You can play by yourself if no one else wants to play with you.

The court wall is 20 feet wide and 16 feet in height. The ball used is called a blue ball at 2.3 ounces.

There are techniques to become a more sufficient player.

Go to www.Handballamerica.com

37

BOWLING

If you know how to bowl, you know this activity is fun and addictive, but with the age of new technologies many of the old bowling alleys are being closed with many modern ones are being built.

This mental and physical game is typically played by 2 people and more.

To play you will need to go to a bowling alley and use their ball or you can bring your own. Bowling Alley shoes are required to maintain the condition of the lanes.

The lane is 60ft in length with 10 pins at the end of the lane. They measure 15 inches in height and are made out of marble.

Your mission is to pick a bowling ball, which weighs between 6 to 16lbs and contain 3 holes: One for you middle finger, one for your ring finger and the other for your thumb.

Rolling the ball down the lane and knocking out all the pins is called a strike.

There are many bowling teams that win prizes. Join one.

www.bowling.com

38

PLAYING INSTRUMENTS

Playing instruments takes skill and practice. The earlier you learn the better you'll be at your choice of instrument as an adult. Many adults have made a career out of using their instrumental talents.

I started playing the drums in High School and I'm pretty good at them now. The favorite instrument in my home is the keyboard.

Instrument categories: Percussion, Brass, Keyboards, Wind, Stringed and Electronic.

My next venture is to learn how to play the Harp. I just can't get enough of the beautiful sounds it makes. Do you have an instrument?

39

<u>BOARDGAMES</u>

Even though this is a sitting down recreation, our hands and mind is always at work. The other benefit of this recreation is that you get to spend time with your loved ones.

One of my favorite board games are Scrabble, checkers, backgammon, monopoly, Life and a new one which is fun bible learning called the Believers Race, visit the website, www.believersrace.com.

Board games could easily be completed in an hour. If you play for 3 hours you know that you'll be exhausted or excited. This depends if you're winning or not.

Board games were here before video games and they're not going anywhere.

40

<u>CHILDREN & PETS</u>

Playing with your children and pets if you have them creates lasting memories.

I have 5 children and they are so active that I sometimes have to tell them to calm down. Children have an abundance of energy.

My children and I go to the neighborhood park, amusement parks, ride our bikes, play video games and wrestle at times.

I put this recreation last because some of us don't take time out for their family. Children are young just for a little while and whatever memory they have in their past they will remember.

The stories of our youth are told to our children and grand children. My children are loaded with questions about what I did as a child.

My pets are many. I believe in sanitizing all the time. I have cats, dogs and parrots. They are our family and we love them and play with them daily.

Enjoy your life and take part in what amuses you. You are only here for a short time. I stress that, because of the day and age we live in now. Don't take life so seriously, but reap the rewards and <u>live</u>. Do Something.

The Pen Moves is a company created by Tanisha Cook to showcase her writings in the area of fiction and non-fiction books, poems, song writing, plays and movie scripts.

Tanisha gets her gifts from the Most High and her ministry background is not the typical one. She was drawn to the ministry after a traumatic time in her life back in March of 1998. She became totally demon possessed. The events are told in her book called

"Demon Possession: It can Happen to You"

Through Tanisha's triumphs and mighty deliverance by the hands of Avi (Father), she has been set free.

Since that day, she has graduated with a certification in Evangelism from the Bible Church of Christ Theological Institute in Bronx,

New York which is her home town. She attended Medgar Evers College in Brooklyn for Language Arts and ordained Pastor alongside her husband Pastor Clyde Cook by Mt. Calvary III Deliverance Outreach, School of the Prophets in Orange, New Jersey.

Better Life Ministries in New Jersey is where she presides over the women. Tanisha believes that women should come together as sisters, learning and teaching each other, because women can teach young women how to be true women of Elohim (God) Titus 2:3-5

www.ingramcontent.com/pod-product-compliance
Lightning Source LLC
Chambersburg PA
CBHW021302280526
45784CB00005B/2473